MW01206573

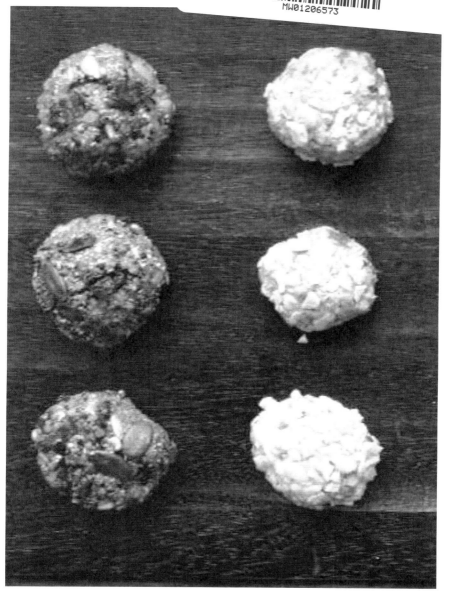

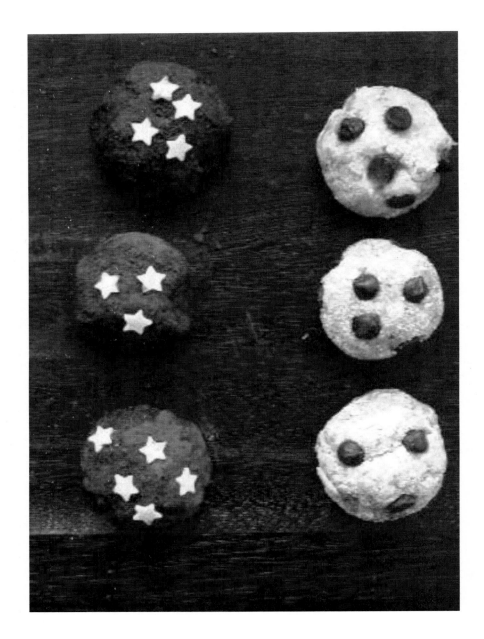

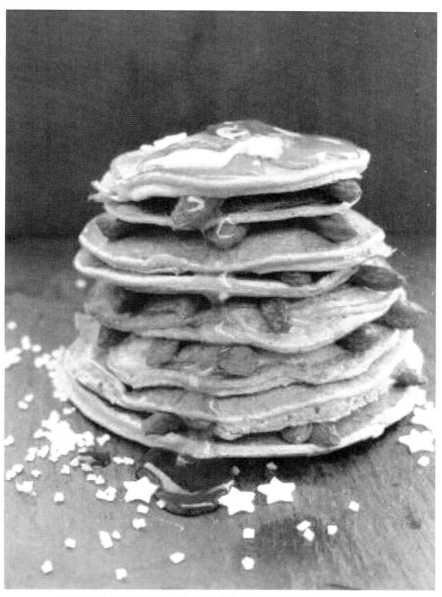

ITEM RECOMMENDATIONS

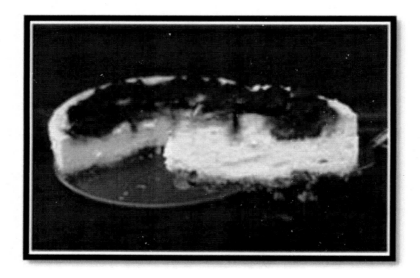

This book contains 27 scrumptious plans made with protein powder.

Baking with protein powder is a pattern that has detonated in the beyond couple of years. Since so many of us have protein powder in our kitchen cabinets, we are normally inquisitive to know how else we can manage it.

I used to imagine that I could basically trade the flour with protein powder in any formula and it would supernaturally change into a tasty high protein creation.

Boy was I wrong....

The outcome was a dull, wipe like catastrophe that even my canine wouldn't eat.

There are heaps of plans online that incorporate protein powder. Yet, one thing that has consistently put me off is the requirement for abnormal and great sorts that I'd never known about. I disdain topping off my cabinets with mass packs of
fixings that I'll just at any point use once.

For this explanation, you will just need three sorts of protein powder to make the plans in this book: unflavoured whey, vanilla whey and pea protein powder. (Indeed, you don't actually require vanilla whey as it's not difficult to make from unflavoured whey - you simply add a little vanilla concentrate and sweetener.)

You may be asking why I didn't pick chocolate whey, as the vast majority will have this in their pantries. The explanation is straightforward: I am yet to find a chocolate-enhanced whey that is adequate. An unfortunate chocolate flavor can demolish your baking, so it's vastly improved to utilize unflavoured whey with a little decent quality cocoa powder and sugar added.

I want to believe that you appreciate making and eating the treats in this book as much as I did.

Let me know how you get on.

PROTEIN BAKING MYTHS

You can swap flour for protein powder

No!

Think about it - flour is a grain, while whey (the most widely recognized kind of protein powder) is a dairy product.

For this explanation, whey will act distinctively when it responds with different fixings in the oven.

Whey goes rubbery and dry when baked

This can be valid, particularly assuming you supplant flour with whey in any recipe.

BUT it doesn't need to be like this. Assuming you include a few extra 'sodden' fixings, similar to coconut oil or yam, they will total out this dryness.

Plant-based protein powders are easier to bake with

This is valid - the majority of the heated plans in this book incorporate pea protein rather than whey. It's only doubtful to bring about a dry, rubbery fiasco when baked.

Protein treats will never taste as good as the real thing

I dissent - give the Cheesecake a shot p12 or the Bounty Bars on p10 and ideally you will feel the same.

RECIPE NOTES

- *all eggs are medium*
- *any kind of milk can be used (macros are based on semi-skimmed cows milk)*
- *any kind of sugar or sweetener can be used (macros are based on using a low-calorie sweetener rather than sugar)*
- *all chocolate is dark minimum 70% cocoa solids*
- *all US imperial measurements are approximate - use the*
- *metric measurements for best results*
- *all macros are approximate and are intended as a guideline only*

PROTEIN

ROCKY ROAD BROWNIES

MAKES 12 BROWNIES

20 MINS PREP
2-3 HOURS CHILLING TIME

INGREDIENTS

125g/1¼ cup/5 scoops unflavoured whey protein

2 tbsp cocoa powder

50g/½ cup fine oats

50g/½ cup goji berries

35g/¼ cup slashed nuts

1 tbsp sugar/sugar 3

tbsp coconut oil

50g/1¾oz dull chocolate

100ml/7 tbsp bubbling

water

15g/½oz smaller than usual marshmallows (optional)

METHOD

1. Add the goji berries and sugar/sugar into a heatproof bowl along with the high temp water. Mix and pass on to douse while you set up the remainder of the ingredients.

2. Melt the coconut oil and dim chocolate together in a little pot on an extremely low hotness. Leave to cool.

3. Prepare the dry fixings: add the whey protein, cocoa powder, fine oats and cleaved nuts into a huge bowl and blend well.

4. Once the goji berries/boiling water and chocolate/coconut oil combinations have cooled, add them both into the enormous bowl with the dry fixings. Blend well.

5. Pour the combination into a brownie plate fixed with greaseproof paper.

6. Push the small scale marshmallows into the highest point of the combination and chill in the refrigerator for 2 - 3 hours.

7. Remove from the cooler and cut into 12 pieces.

Recipe notes:

- *You can add whatever fillings you want to this recipe – whey protein crispies, shortbread pieces and dried fruit all work well.*

- *Be sure to include some pistachios as they look great when the brownies are sliced.*

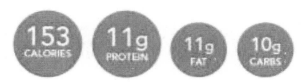

MACROS (PER BROWNIE)

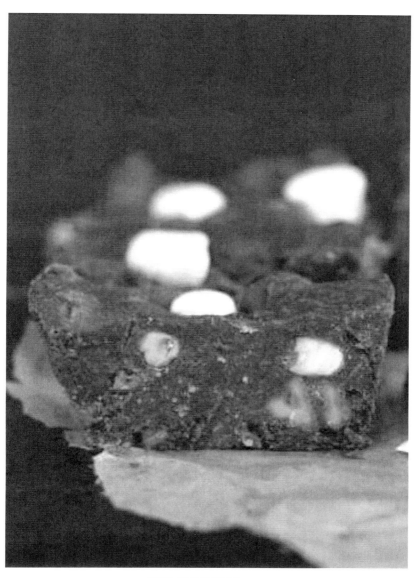

PROTEIN
BOUNTY BAR

MAKES 4 BARS

20 MINS PREP
45 MINS CHILLING TIME

INGREDIENTS

50g/½ cup/2 scoops vanilla whey protein

4 tbsp milk

20g/¾oz dessicated coconut, in addition to some extra for

tidying 2 tbsp coconut oil

40g/1½oz dim chocolate

METHOD

1. Melt the coconut oil and save to the side a teaspoonful for later in the formula. Blend the rest in with the vanilla whey and dessicated coconut.

2. Slowly add the milk. When the consistency of the combination is tacky however not excessively wet, shape into 4 bars on a sheet of greaseproof paper with some extra dried up coconut sprinkled over it to make the combination more straightforward to handle.

3. Put the bars in the cooler for around 30 minutes to set.

4. Meanwhile, liquefy the chocolate with the leftover coconut oil (add the coconut oil to the dish first so the chocolate doesn't burn).

5. Take the bars out of the refrigerator and dunk in the softened chocolate.

6. Return them to the ice chest until the chocolate sets (this should take around 15 minutes).

Recipe notes:

- *You can leave out the coconut oil from this recipe and save 60 calories and 7g of fat per bar. However, the texture won't be quite as Bounty-*

like.

- *If you are short of time or very hungry, you can also put the bars in the freezer to set. Just keep an eye on them so they don't freeze completely.*

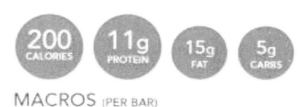

MACROS (PER BAR)

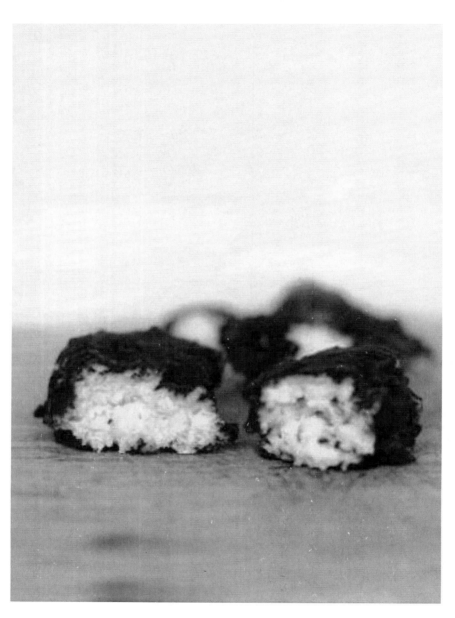

PROTEIN

BLUEBERRY CHEESECAKE

SERVES 8

20 MINS PREP
30 - 40 MINS BAKING

INGREDIENTS

100g/3½oz natural product and

nut blend 500g/17½oz 0% fat

Greek yogurt 250g/8¾oz vanilla

quark

25g/¼ cup/1 scoop vanilla whey protein

2 eggs

100g/3½oz blueberries

1 tbsp sugar/sweetener

METHOD

1. Preheat the broiler to 160°C/320°F.

2. Place the organic product and nut blend in a food processor and mix. When the blend has turned into a fine however marginally tacky powder, press it down into the lower part of a 20cm/8" free base non stick cake tin.

3. Meanwhile, combine as one the Greek yogurt, vanilla quark, vanilla whey and eggs. Spread this blend over the base.

4. Bake in the broiler until the highest point of the cheesecake is recently cooked. This should accept 30 - 40 minutes.

5. Meanwhile, place the blueberries in a pan along with the sugar/sugar and hotness delicately until the berries become delicate. Utilizing a spoon or fork,

burst the berries and mix until the blend thickens a bit. Eliminate from the container and let the blend cool.

6. Once the cheesecake is done, eliminate from the stove and let it cool.

7. Once both have chilled off, pour the blueberry besting over the base.

8. Slice into 8 pieces and serve.

Recipe notes:

- *If you can't find vanilla quark, you can use unflavoured quark with a teaspoon of vanilla extract and a teaspoon of sugar/sweetener.*
- *Take care not to overcook the cheesecake.*
- *Remove it from the oven as soon as the top stops wobbling. It will taste better if slightly undercooked than if overcooked.*

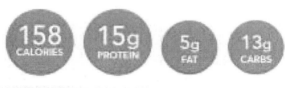

MACROS (PER SLICE)

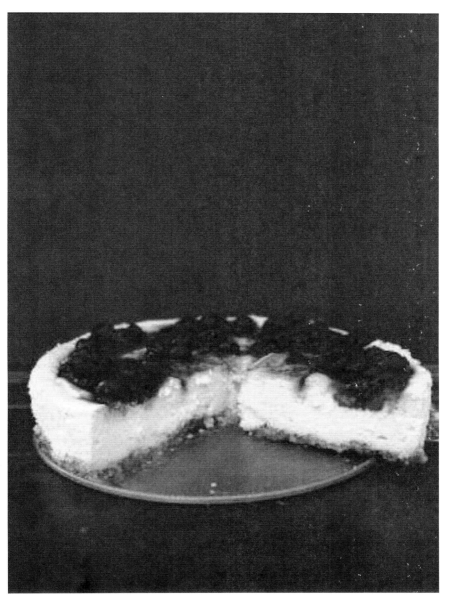

CHOCOLATE PROTEIN TRUFFLES

MAKES 10 TRUFFLES

20 MINS PREP
1 HOUR + CHILLING TIME

INGREDIENTS

25g/1oz dim chocolate

2 tbsp coconut oil

50g/½ cup/2 scoops unflavoured whey protein

1 tsp cocoa powder (+ extra for rolling)

1 tsp sugar/sweetener

3 tbsp milk

METHOD

1. Melt the coconut oil and dull chocolate together cautiously in a pot on an extremely low hotness. When dissolved, let the combination cool completely.

2. Once cooled, join with different fixings in general. Blend well and leave in the ice chest for at minimum an hour.

3. Now for the muddled piece - spoon out a teaspoonful of the combination and roll into a ball, utilizing a little cocoa powder to cover.

4. Repeat for every one of the 10 truffles.

Recipe notes:

- *For extra creaminess and vitamins, try adding a ripe avocado into the mixture at step 2.*
- *You can flavour the truffles with orange or peppermint oil.....or even some rum.*

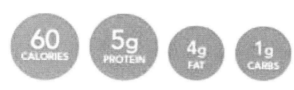

MACROS (PER TRUFFLE)

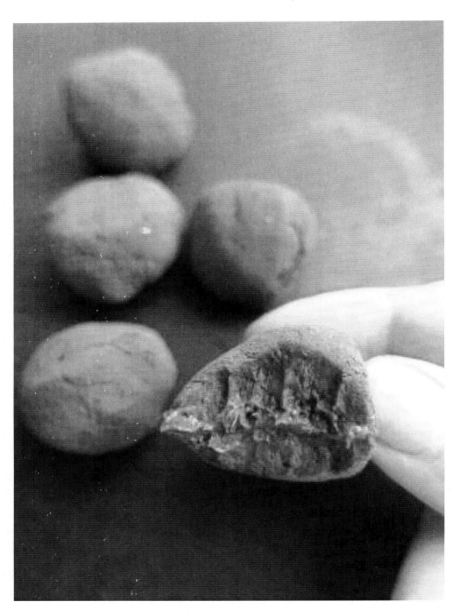

PROTEIN ROCHER

MAKES 14

INGREDIENTS

50g/½ cup fine oats

100g/3½oz whey protein crispies

75g/¾ cup/3 scoops vanilla whey protein

100g/½ cup coconut oil

200g/7oz nut butter

8 squashed malted milk rolls

100g/3½oz dull chocolate

METHOD

1. Melt the coconut oil in the microwave or on the hob. Save to the side a tablespoonful for step 6.

2. Once liquefied and cooled, empty the coconut oil into an enormous bowl alongside the other dry fixings: the oats, whey protein crispies, vanilla whey and squashed biscuits.

3. Add in the peanut butter and mix until everything is combined.

4. Place the bowl in the refrigerator for 15 minutes to set.

5. Once chilled, eliminate from the ice chest and roll into 14 balls.

6. Carefully liquefy the chocolate and remaining coconut oil.

7. Coat the balls in the chocolate/oil blend and spot them back in the cooler for an additional 15 minutes, until the chocolate has set.

Recipe notes:

- *This recipe was inspired by a GoNutrition recipe of which I made a video....it was simply too good not to include in the book. It could be easily adapted to lower the fat and calorie content by using less coconut oil and by leaving out the biscuits. The result would be less crunchy but still a yummy treat.*

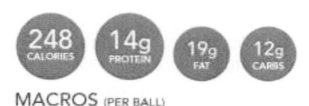

MACROS (PER BALL)

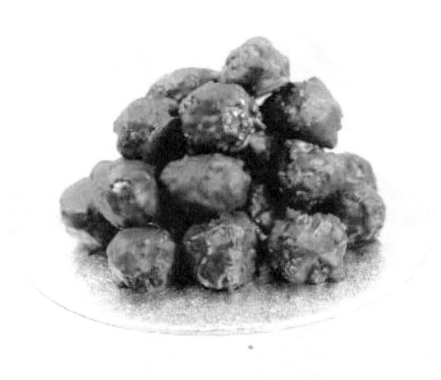

PEANUT CHOCOLATE SWIRL

PROTEIN FLAPJACKS by Gymster

MAKES 8

30 MINS PREP
15 MINS BAKING
1.5 HOURS CHILLING TIME

INGREDIENTS

200g/7oz peanut butter

100g/3½oz honey

250g/9oz oats

100g/1 cup/4 scoops vanilla whey protein

1 tbsp coconut oil

150ml/2/3 cup milk

150g/51/3oz dim chocolate

METHOD

1. Preheat the stove to 200°C/390°F.

2. Melt the coconut oil. Combine as one with the honey and a big part of the peanut butter. Ensure everything is dissolved appropriately and in fluid form.

3. In a different bowl, join the vanilla whey and the milk. Once mixed, include the coconut oil/honey/peanut butter blend along with the oats.

4. Flatten the combination into a baking plate and prepare in the broiler for 15 minutes. Once done, eliminate from the broiler and pass on to cool slightly.

5. Meanwhile, soften the dim chocolate and staying peanut butter independently (this should be possible in the hot stove in two separate dishes).

6. Firstly, pour the dissolved chocolate over the hotcake base and spread until covered.

7. Secondly, pour the liquefied peanut butter over the dissolved chocolate and, utilizing the rear of a spoon, blend it around a little to make swirls.

8. Let the pancakes cool for 30 minutes and spot in the refrigerator for a further hour.

9. Once cooled, cut into 8 slices.

Recipe notes:

- *This recipe belongs to my friend Mark Runza. Mark's app, Gymster, has over 170 great recipes like this one. You can download it from the App store and it's available for Android too.*

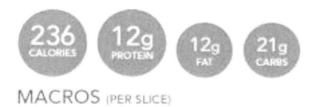

MACROS (PER SLICE)

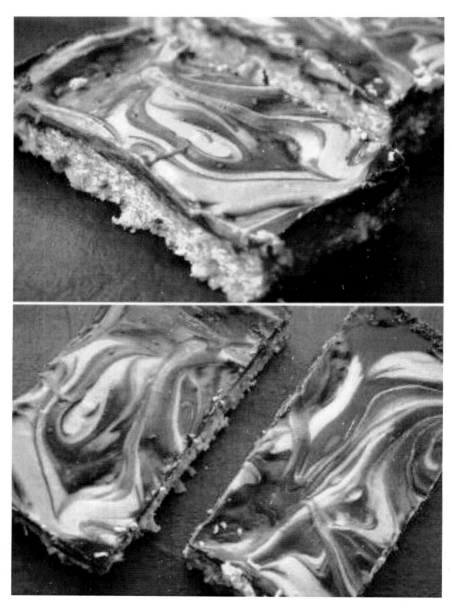

NO BAKE PROTEIN

GRANOLA COOKIES

MAKES 5

5 MINS PREP
30 MINS CHILLING TIME

INGREDIENTS

50g/1¾oz granola

25g/¼ cup/1 scoop unflavoured whey protein

2 tbsp nut butter

2 tbsp milk

1 tablespoon coconut flour

METHOD

1. Add the granola, whey protein, coconut flour and peanut butter into a mixing bowl and gradually add in the milk until you get the right texture (i.e. wet enough so that everything sticks together but not too wet).

2. Mix everything together and, utilizing your hands, separate into 5 balls.

3. Flatten each ball into a round treat shape and put in the cooler to chill for 30 minutes.

Recipe notes:

- *This recipe is so simple and quick.....because the granola is already baked, the finished cookies are crunchy without the need for baking.*

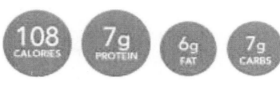

MACROS (PER COOKIE)

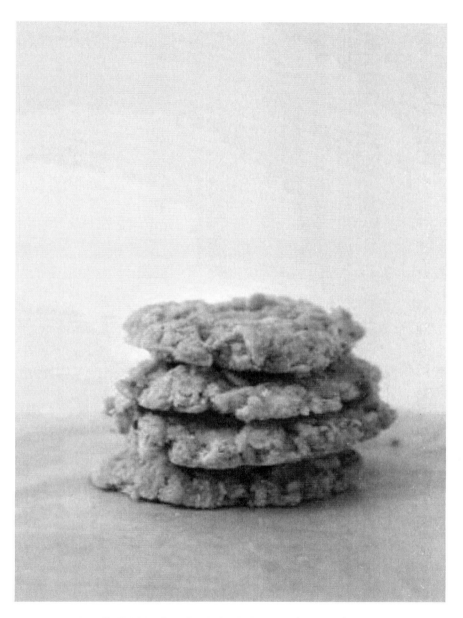

PROTEIN BIRTHDAY CAKE

MAKES 12 SLICES

20 MINS PREP
20 MINS BAKING

INGREDIENTS

50g/½ cup/2 scoops unflavoured whey protein powder

2 tsp vanilla extract

3 eggs

150ml/½ cup dissolved coconut

oil 100g/3½oz ground almonds

5 tbsp sugar/sugar 6

tbsp cocoa powder

100ml/7 tbsp water

1 tsp baking powder for the icing:

100g/3½oz vanilla quark

25g/¼ cup/1 scoop vanilla whey protein

1 tbsp cocoa powder

METHOD

1. Preheat the broiler to 170°C/340°F. Line the foundation of a 20cm/8" free base non stick cake tin with greaseproof paper and utilize a tablespoon or so of the

dissolved coconut oil to lube both the paper and the sides of the tin.

2. Using an electric whisk, beat together the eggs and sugar/sugar in an enormous blending bowl. Once foamy, gradually beat in the leftover coconut oil (ensure it has cooled totally beforehand).

3. Using a wooden spoon, cautiously overlay in the excess cake ingredients.

4. Pour the blend into the cake tin and prepare for 20 minutes, or until a mixed drink stick confesses all with the exception of a couple of chocolate crumbs.

5. Remove from the stove and pass on the cake to cool in its tin.

6. Meanwhile, make the icing: utilizing an electric whisk, consolidate the vanilla quark with the vanilla whey and cocoa powder.

7. Once the cake has cooled, cover in icing and serve.

Recipe notes:

- *This recipe was inspired by Nigella's chocolate olive oil cake. As with Nigella's version, you can swap the almond flour for regular plain flour (use 75g) which will result in it being lighter and more 'cake'-like.*
- *The cake would also be perfect with some icing sugar sprinkled over the top in place of the quark-based icing.*

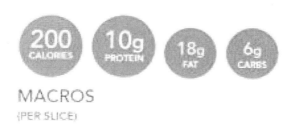

MACROS
(PER SLICE)

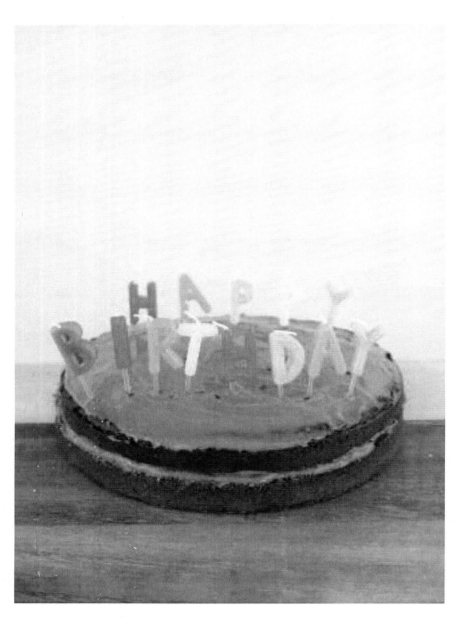

PROTEIN SNICKERS

MAKES 6

INGREDIENTS

100g/1 cup/4 scoops vanilla whey protein

4 tbsp coconut flour (in addition to some extra for

tidying) 100ml/7 tbsp milk

6 medjool dates

20g/¾oz hacked blended nuts

1 tsp salted caramel seasoning

60g/2oz dim chocolate

1 tbsp coconut oil

METHOD

1. Add the vanilla whey and coconut flour into a large mixing bowl and gradually add the milk until you get the right texture of dough (i.e. wet enough so that it sticks together but not too sticky to handle).

2. Separate into 6 similarly measured balls and afterward level into bar shapes utilizing your hands. Pass on the bars in the refrigerator to cool a little.

3. To make the fixing: eliminate the stones from the medjool dates and mix along with the salted caramel enhancing in a food processor to make a paste.

4. Spoon the glue over the highest point of each bar and press some cleaved blended nuts into the top.

5. Using a little pan, cautiously soften the chocolate and coconut oil together.

6. Remove the bars from the cooler and cover in chocolate. Return them into

the refrigerator to set, which should take a further 30 minutes.

Recipe notes:

- *The salted caramel flavouring is optional, but highly recommended. You can also use it to make the salted caramel protein balls on page 36.*

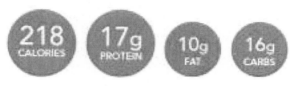

MACROS (PER BAR)

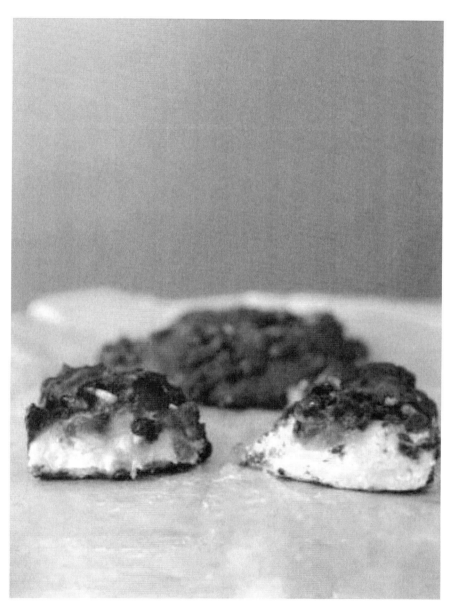

CHOCOLATE PROTEIN

LAVA CAKE

SERVES 2

5 MINS PREP
3 - 5 MINS BAKING

INGREDIENTS

25g/¼ cup/1 scoop unflavoured whey protein

1 tbsp cocoa powder

1 egg

1 tbsp sugar/sugar 1

tbsp ground almonds 2

tbsp coconut oil

2 tbsp milk

METHOD

1. Preheat the stove to 180°C/350°F. Line the lower part of a ramekin (or two, assuming that you can track down tiny ones) with greaseproof paper - follow around the outside of the base and slice with scissors to make it fit.

2. Melt the coconut oil and utilize a teaspoonful to lube the sides of the ramekin(s).

3. Mix the leftover coconut oil with every one of different fixings in a mixing bowl. Once mixed, fill the ramekin and heat in the hot oven.

4. After 3 minutes, verify whether the top and sides of the cake are completely cooked. Provided that this is true, it's ready.

5. Using a blade, separate the sides of the cake away from the ramekin. Place a topsy turvy plate over the ramekin and afterward flip both. The cake ought

to ideally tumble down onto the plate intact.

6. Peel off the greaseproof paper and serve.

Recipe notes:

- *Don't be tempted to leave out the greaseproof paper – the bottom of the cake will stick and it will be impossible to get out.*
- *This recipe would also make a fantastic mug cake – microwave it for around 30 seconds – 1 minute.*

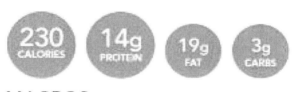

MACROS (PER SERVING)

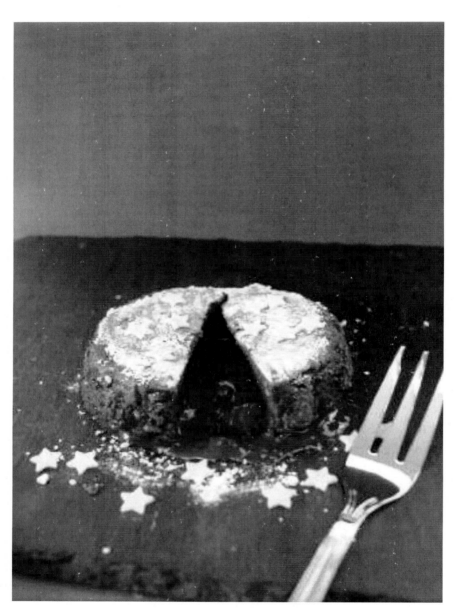

PROTEIN SCONES

MAKES 5

10 MINS PREP
15 MINS BAKING

INGREDIENTS

125g/4½oz wholemeal self-raising flour (in addition to extra for

cleaning) 50g/1¾oz salted butter

25g/¼ cup/1 scoop vanilla or unflavoured whey protein (see notes)

70ml/1/3 cup milk

1 egg (discretionary, for brushing over the top)

METHOD

1. Preheat the oven to 180°C/350°F. Line a baking tray with some greaseproof paper.

2. Mix together the flour, margarine, whey protein and milk to get a delicate dough.

3. Turn on to a floured work surface and ply gently. Search level until around 2cm thick. Utilize a 5cm/2in shaper to get rid of rounds and put on the baking plate. Gently massage together the remainder of the batter and stamp out more scones to utilize it all up.

4. Brush the highest points of the scones with the beaten egg. Heat for around 15 minutes until very much risen and golden.

Recipe notes:

- *For sweet scones, use vanilla whey protein or unflavoured whey plus a little vanilla essence and sugar/sweetener.*

- *For savoury scones, use unflavoured whey (a pinch of sugar or sweetener will take away the bitterness of the flour). You could even top with some grated cheese.*

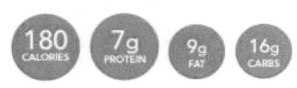

MACROS (PER SCONE)

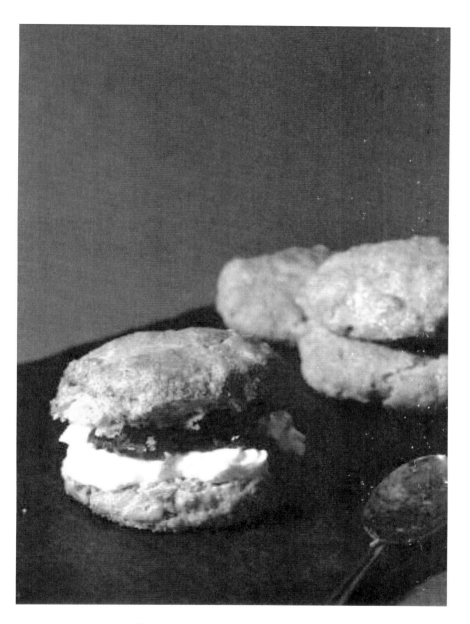

SWEET POTATO

PROTEIN BROWNIES

MAKES 8 BROWNIES

5 MINS PREP
30 MINS BAKING

INGREDIENTS

1 medium measured yam (around 300g/10oz in weight)

100g/3½oz nut butter

25g/¼ cup/1 scoop unflavoured whey protein

2 tsp cocoa powder

1 tsp sugar/sugar 25g/1oz

chocolate, melted

METHOD

1. Prick the yam done with a fork and microwave on high for 8 to 10 minutes, turning once. Eliminate, check that within is delicate and let it cool.

2. Preheat the broiler to 180°C/350°F and oil or line a brownie tin with greaseproof paper.

3. Once cooled, scoop out within the potato and pound until smooth. Include the peanut butter, whey protein, cocoa powder, sugar/sugar and dissolved chocolate. Combine everything as one until smooth.

4. Pour the blend into the brownie tin. Utilizing a fork or spoon, spread the blend along the entire of the tin, making it level.

5. Bake for around 20 minutes, until the top is well cooked.

6. Remove the brownie tin from the stove, let it cool for a couple of moments and afterward cautiously cut into 8 pieces.

Recipe notes:

- *Be sure to mash the sweet potato well, breaking it up completely. The last thing you want to find in your brownie is a piece of sweet potato*
- *You can also peel and cube the sweet potato and cook it in the microwave or in boiling water.*

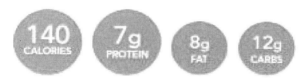

MACROS (PER BROWNIE)

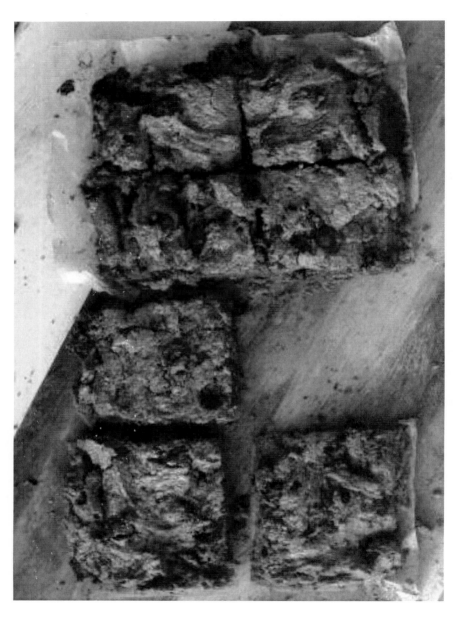

WONGKA'S APPLE,

RAISIN & CINNAMON EGG ROLLS

MAKES 4 ROLLS

15 MINS PREP
45 MINS COOKING TIME

INGREDIENTS

2 apples, center eliminated and

slashed 2 tsp coconut oil

1 square lavash bread

4 tbsp water

2 tsp sugar/sweetener

1 tsp cinnamon

30g/1oz raisins

1 tsp honey

60g/2oz medium fat cream

cheddar 1 egg

2 tbsp milk

METHOD

1. Heat up 1 tsp of the coconut oil in a pot and tenderly cook the hacked apples. After around 5 minutes, add the raisins, cinnamon, sugar/sugar, water and honey. Tenderly stew until the apples have relaxed - this should take around 10 minutes.

2. Cut the lavash bread into 4 bits. Spread around 15g of the cheddar on each, along with a fourth of the apple filling. Fold every one into a cylinder.

3. Beat the egg and include the milk. Empty this blend into a shallow dish

and plunge in the rolls. Pass on every one to splash for a couple minutes.

4. Heat up the excess coconut oil and fry the rolls on high hotness for around 4 minutes, or until brilliant brown.

Recipe notes:

- *This recipe is by my friend Willy Wong. Take a look at his Instagram (@willy_w0ngka) for loads more great recipes.*
- *Lavash bread is ideal for this recipe as it is rectangular (Willy is a fan of a brand called Joseph's). If you can't get hold of it, you can use any kind of wrap or tortilla.*

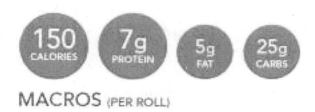

MACROS (PER ROLL)

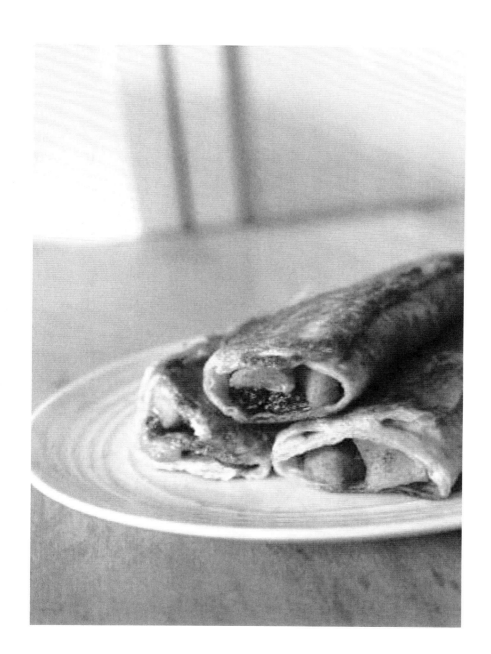

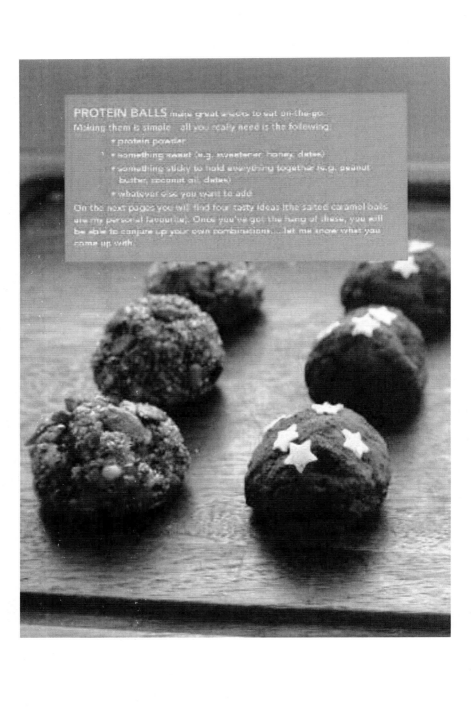

PROTEIN BALLS make great snacks to eat on-the-go.
Making them is simple – all you really need is the following:

- protein powder
- something sweet (e.g. sweetener, honey, dates)
- something sticky to hold everything together (e.g. peanut butter, coconut oil, dates)
- whatever else you want to add

On the next pages you will find four tasty ideas (the salted caramel balls are my personal favourite). Once you've got the hang of these, you will be able to conjure up your own combinations... let me know what you come up with.

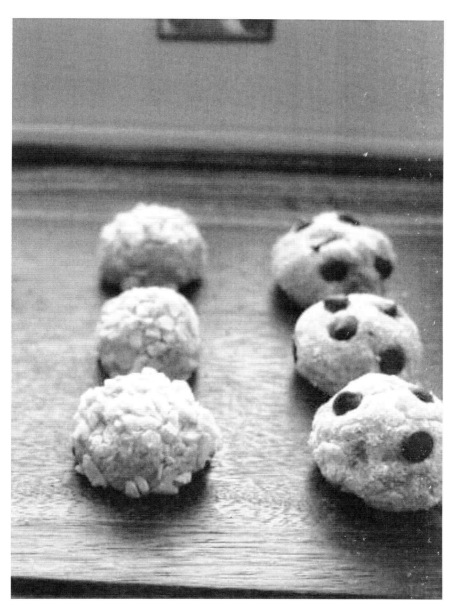

SALTED CARAMEL PROTEIN

BALLS

MAKES 6 BALLS

5 MINS PREP

INGREDIENTS

6 medjool dates

50g/½ cup/2 scoops unflavoured whey protein

2 tbsp water

1/2 tsp salted caramel enhancing (discretionary)

20g/¾oz slashed nuts

METHOD

1. Carefully cook the cleaved nuts in a skillet (no requirement for any oil) until carmelized. Keep aside.

2. Remove the stones from the medjool dates and add, along with the whey protein, water and salted caramel seasoning (if utilizing), into a food processor.

3. Blend until completely combined.

4. Divide the combination into 6 balls and roll in the blended nuts to cover.

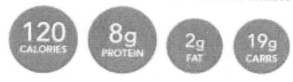

MACROS (PER BALL)

CHOCOLATE CHIP COOKIE

DOUGH
PROTEIN BALLS

MAKES 8 BALLS

5 MINS PREP

INGREDIENTS

50g/½ cup/1 scoop vanilla whey protein

4 tbsp milk

2 piled tbsp (40g) almond

margarine 2 tbsp ground almonds

2 tbsp coconut flour

30g/1oz chocolate chips

METHOD

1. Mix together the vanilla whey, almond spread, ground almonds and coconut flour. Include the milk slowly - you might require somewhat more or minimal less relying upon how runny the almond margarine is. The blend ought to be delicate however not too tacky to even think about dealing with (assuming it turns out to be excessively tacky, essentially add somewhat more of any of the dry fixings or chill in the fridge).

2. Divide into 8 balls and push in the chocolate chips.

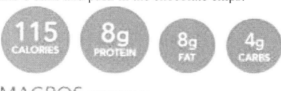

MACROS (PER BALL)

CHOCOLATE GOJI PROTEIN BALLS

MAKES 8 BALLS

10 MINS PREP

INGREDIENTS

25g/1oz coconut oil

25g/1oz dim chocolate

25g/1oz goji berries

1 tsp sugar/sugar

50ml/3 tbsp hot water

50g/½ cup/2 scoops unflavoured whey protein

1 tbsp cocoa powder (in addition to extra for

rolling) 25g/1oz fine oats

METHOD

1. Melt the coconut oil and dim chocolate together in a pan on an extremely low hotness, taking consideration not to consume the chocolate. Leave to cool.

2. Add the boiling water and sugar/sugar to the goji berries and leave for 15 minutes or so to rehydrate the berries.

3. Once both the berries/high temp water and chocolate/coconut oil combinations have cooled, combine as one and add the oats, cocoa powder and vanilla whey.

4. Roll into balls and cover in cocoa powder.

MACROS (PER BALL)

SUPERFOOD PROTEIN BALLS

MAKES 8 BALLS

5 MINS PREP

INGREDIENTS

100g/3½oz cooked quinoa 50g/½

cup/2 scoops vanilla whey 2 tbsp

milk

2 tbsp peanut butter

1 tsp honey

1 tbsp chia seeds

1 tbsp pumpkin/sunflower seeds

1 tbsp dried cranberries

METHOD

1. Mix together the cooked quinoa, vanilla whey, milk, peanut butter and honey until well blended.

2. Shape into 8 balls.

3. Pour out the seeds/cranberries onto a plate and roll around the balls to coat.

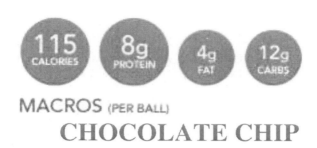

MACROS (PER BALL)

CHOCOLATE CHIP

PROTEIN COOKIES

MAKES 8 MINI COOKIES

10 MINS PREP
10 - 15 MINS BAKING

INGREDIENTS

25g/¼ cup/1 scoop pea protein

½ cup/50g oats

100ml/7 tbsp milk

1 tbsp almond butter

1 tbsp coconut oil,

liquefied 3 tbsp

sugar/sugar 15g/½oz

chocolate chips

METHOD

1. Preheat the broiler to 180°C/350°F. Line a baking plate with greaseproof paper. 2. Join the pea protein, oats, milk, almond margarine, coconut oil and sugar/sugar. Blend well.

3. Spoon the combination onto the baking plate (you ought to have the option to make 8 little treats), straighten and press a few chocolate chips into each cookie.

4. Bake for 10 - 15 minutes, until they are simply cooked.

Recipe notes:

- *Be careful not to overbake the cookies.... they will taste much better undercooked than overcooked.*

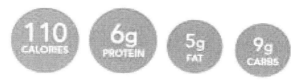

MACROS (PER COOKIE)

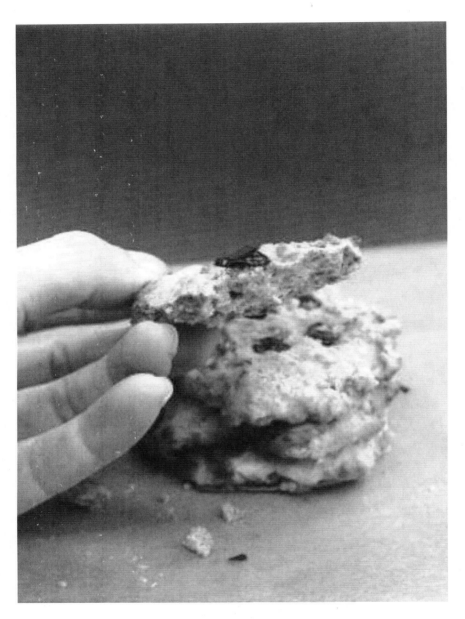

PROTEIN

MINCE PIES

MAKES 12

20 MINS PREP
45 MINS COOKING

INGREDIENTS

for the 'mincemeat':

2 medium apples 1

tbsp coconut oil

150g/5 1/3 oz dried organic

product 1/2 cup water

1 tsp sugar/sugar 1 tsp

vanilla extract

1 tsp ground ginger 1

tsp cinnamon

for the pastry:

50g/½ cup/2 scoops pea protein

100g/3½ wholemeal self-raising flour (in addition to extra for

cleaning) 60g/½ cup ground almonds

150g/5 1/3 oz plain yogurt

2 egg whites

1 tbsp sugar/sweetener

METHOD

1. Firstly make the 'mincemeat': eliminate the centers and slash the apples into little pieces. Liquefy the coconut oil in a little pot and add the apple pieces. Fry for a couple of moments, blending constantly.

2. Add the excess mincemeat fixings and mix. Stew for around 30 minutes, adding more water in the event that the combination starts to dry out.

3. Preheat the broiler to 180°C/350°F and oil a 12-opening biscuit skillet and a different baking tray.

4. Using a food processor, consolidate the baked good fixings until they structure a dough.

5. Tip out onto a gently floured surface and manipulate the mixture until it turns out to be adequately firm to roll.

6. Roll out the batter as slender as conceivable utilizing either your hands or a moving pin. Utilizing a round shaper or a cup, cut out 12 bases and spot them into the lubed biscuit plate. Utilizing a star shaper (or a blade in the event that you don't have one), cut out 12 stars and spot onto the lubed baking tray.

7. Bake for 10 - 15 minutes, or until daintily browned.

8. Remove the mince pie bases from the broiler and spoon in some 'mincemeat' into every one. Put a star on top and serve.

Recipe notes:

- *Depending on how thick the yoghurt you use is (I used Skyr), the pastry may need a little more or less (if you put in too much, just add more of one of the dry ingredients).*
- *The pastry would also make a great pizza base or quiche crust (just add a pinch of sugar/sweetener rather than a tablespoon for a more savoury pastry).*
- *If you have some oranges or lemons handy, a little grated zest in the mincemeat would be lovely. As would a shot of brandy.*

MACROS (PER MINCE PIE)

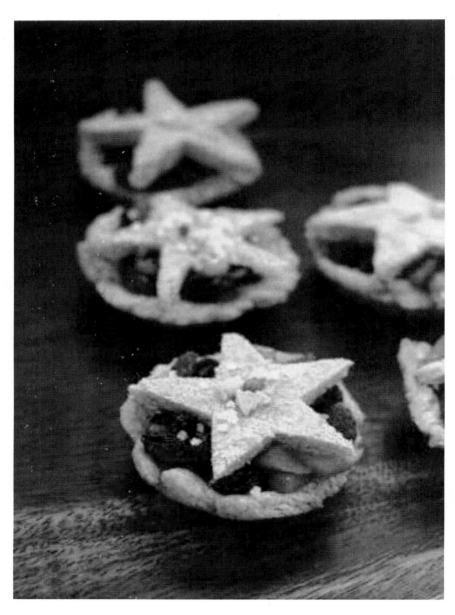

PROTEIN EGGNOG

SERVES 3

INGREDIENTS

250ml/1 cup milk

25g/¼ cup/1 scoop vanilla whey

1 cinnamon stick

½ tsp newly ground nutmeg (in addition to extra for

serving). 2 eggs, separated

1 tbsp sugar/sugar a fix

of rum (optional)

METHOD

1. Add the vanilla whey and milk into a protein shaker and shake well to combine.

2. Pour into a little pot and add the cinnamon stick and nutmeg. Heat delicately - don't bring to the bubble. Eliminate from the hotness not long before it arrives at the purpose in bubbling and leave to steep.

3. Using a handheld whisk, beat the egg yolks and sugar/sugar until consolidated and thick.

4. Combine this egg yolk blend with the whey combination and mix until joined and smooth. Add the rum, if utilizing, and leave in the ice chest to cool.

5. Before serving, beat the egg whites with an electric race until delicate pinnacles structure. Tenderly overlay this into the eggnog.

6. Serve with ground nutmeg on top.

Recipe notes:

- *Be careful not to overheat the whey, it will curdle.*
- *Eggnog is traditionally made with cream, which tastes great but makes the calorie and fat count shoot up. You can add some double cream to this recipe if you want, it will taste amazing.*
- *The shot of rum is optional but highly recommended.*

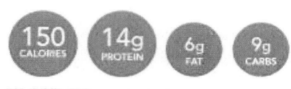

MACROS (PER SERVING)

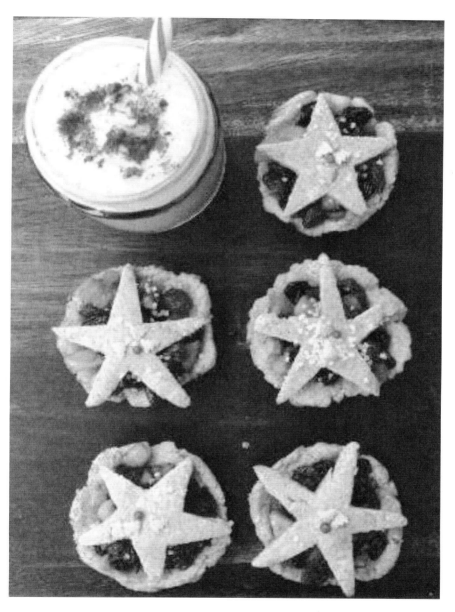

CHRISTMAS PROTEIN PANCAKES

MAKES 8 PANCAKES
SERVES 2

5 MINS PREP
10 MINS COOKING

INGREDIENTS

25g/¼ cup/1 scoop unflavoured whey

25g/¼ cup/1 scoop fine oats

1 medium ready

banana 1 egg + 2 egg

whites a modest

bunch of spinach

1 tsp baking powder

2 tsp coconut oil

METHOD

1. Place every one of the fixings with the exception of the coconut oil in a food processor and blend them together.

2. Heat half of the coconut oil up in a skillet on low-medium hotness and cautiously spoon in 4 circles of batter.

3. Flip over once sautéed (this should just require a couple of moments) and eliminate from the container once the second side is done.

4. Add the excess oil and repeat.

Recipe notes:

- *Who needs green food colouring when you have spinach?? You won't even be able to taste it.*

- *You can of course leave the spinach out or, if it's nowhere near Christmas time, call them 'Hulk' pancakes.*

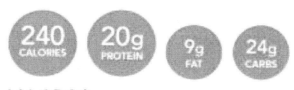

MACROS (PER SERVING)

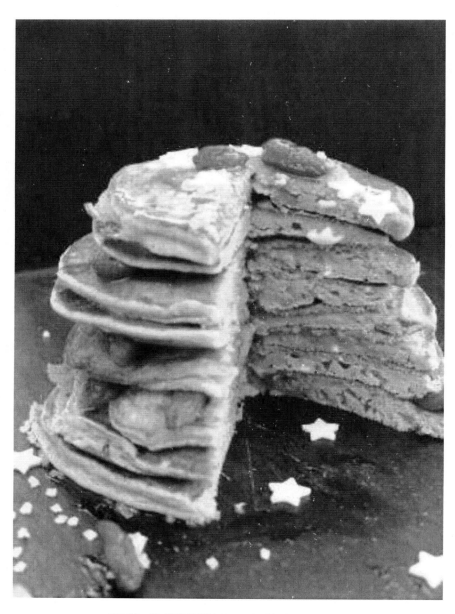

PROTEIN BISCUITS

MAKES 5 BISCUITS

5 MINS PREP
10 - 15 MINS BAKING

INGREDIENTS

100g/1 cup ground almonds (in addition to some extra for

tidying) 25g/¼ cup/1 scoop pea protein

1 tbsp water

5 medjool dates, stones

eliminated 1 egg white

METHOD

1. Heat the broiler to 170°C/340°F. Line a baking plate with some greaseproof paper.

2. Put each of the fixings in a food processor and blend completely until the dates have totally separated and the combination has turned into a firm dough.

3. Sprinkle some ground almonds on a spotless surface and level the mixture, utilizing your hands, until it is around a large portion of a centimeter thick.

4. Using a cutout, cut out 5 shapes (you will presumably need to shape the last one utilizing your hands) and put on the baking tray.

5. Bake for 10 - 15 minutes, or until the rolls have become brilliant brown.

Recipe notes:

- *Anything with ground nuts in will burn very easily, so be sure to bake at a low oven temperature and keep an eye on the biscuits.*
- *If you don't want to use expensive ground almonds for dusting, any kind*

of flour will do.

- *If you want to use these as tree decorations as I have, use a cocktail stick to make a hole in each biscuit before baking for the silver thread to fit through. Decorate with some instant icing (not included in the macros sadly..).*

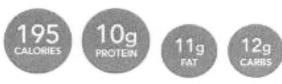

MACROS (PER BISCUIT)

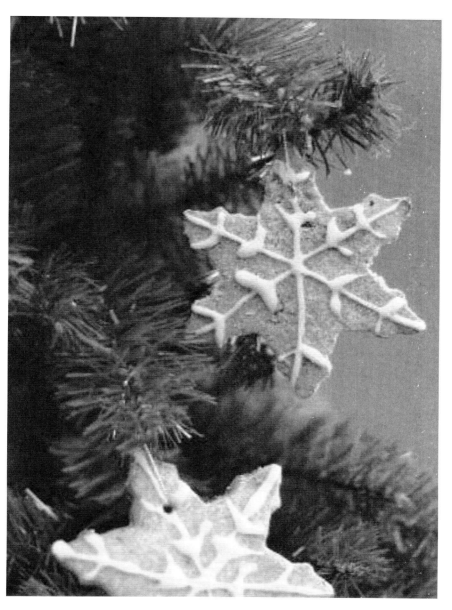

PROTEIN BANANA BREAD

MAKES 10 SLICES

INGREDIENTS

4 medium bananas

50g/½ cup/2 scoops unflavoured whey

100g/1 cup ground almonds

50g/½ cup coconut flour

1 tsp baking powder

60g/½ cup pecan pieces

2 eggs

METHOD

1. Preheat the broiler to 180°C/350°F. Oil a 20cm/8in portion tin.

2. Combine three of the bananas with different fixings in general. Pound the banana generally (don't stress over getting it totally smooth - the knots will taste great) yet ensure all the other things is blended.

3. Spoon the combination into the portion tin. Cut the excess banana into two lengthways and spot over the top.

4. Bake for 50 - 60 minutes.

Recipe notes:

- *This is a flourless recipe, which means that the result is a little softer and heavier than regular banana bread. You could always replace some of the ground almonds with plain flour for a more 'cake'-like texture.*

- *The riper the bananas are, the sweeter the finished banana bread will be.*
- *The addition of the walnut pieces is highly recommended....however, if you leave them out, you will save 40 calories and 4g of fat per slice.*

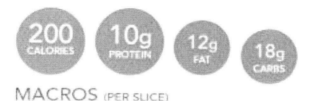

MACROS (PER SLICE)

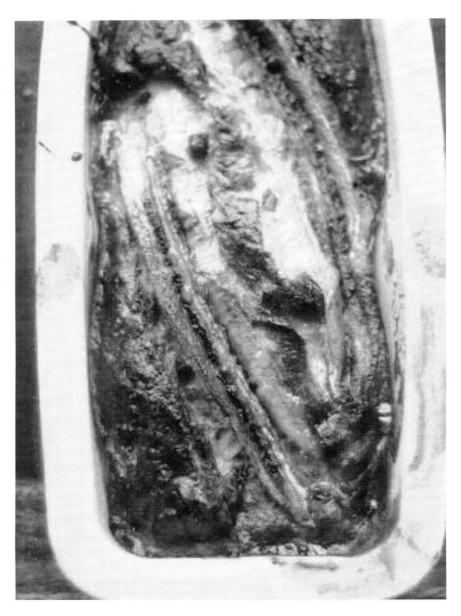

PROTEIN

S'MORES IN A MUG

MAKES 1

10 MINS PREP
5 MINS COOKING

INGREDIENTS

for the hot chocolate:

25g/¼ cup/1 scoop unflavoured whey

70ml/1/3 cup milk

1 tbsp cashew

margarine 1 tbsp cocoa

1 tbsp sugar/sweetener

for the cookie:

4 tbsp ground almonds (in addition to some extra for

cleaning) 1 tsp pea protein

1 medjool date, stone eliminated

1 tsp egg white

6 smaller than expected marshmallows

METHOD

1. Firstly, make the treat: place the treat fixings into a food processor and blend until a mixture is framed. Eliminate the batter from the food processor and keep aside.

2. Next, place all of the hot cocoa fixings into the food processor (no compelling reason to clean it) and blend until a thick chocolaty syrup is shaped. Empty this out into a mug.

3. Gently heat the hot cocoa blend in the microwave, being extremely mindful so as not to allow it to arrive at limit (heat up in 10 second bursts).

4. Shape the bread roll batter into a round shape and put on top of the hot cocoa. Push in the smaller than normal marshmallows and spot under a hot barbecue for a couple of moments, until the roll is gently toasted and the marshmallows are melted.

Recipe notes:

- *This is a very indulgent treat for one. The protein hot chocolate is very good on its own and has only 235 calories, 26g protein, 12g fat and 12g carbs.*

- *Be careful not to overheat the hot chocolate; the whey will curdle.*

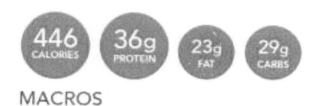

MACROS

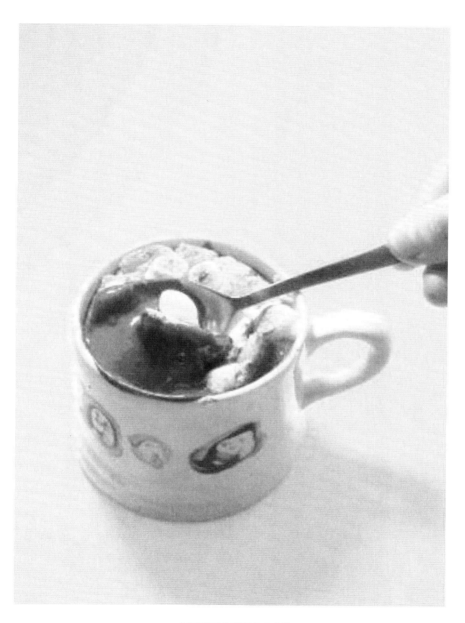

WONGKA'S

SALTED CHILI-CHOCOANANA BITES

MAKES 16

15 MINS PREP
1.5 HOURS CHILLING TIME

INGREDIENTS

1 ready banana

50g/½ cup/2 scoops vanilla whey protein

80g/1 cup oats

2 tbsp almond butter

to coat:

100g/3½oz dim chocolate

1 tbsp coconut oil

ocean salt

red bean stew flakes

METHOD

1. Mash the banana and join with 60g of the oats, the vanilla whey and almond butter.

2. Sprinkle the leftover oats over a plate and use them as a cleaning to assist you with molding the blend into a major square shape. Freeze for 1 - 2 hours.

3. Melt the chocolate and coconut oil together.

4. Cut the banana/oat combination into squares and plunge every one into the chocolate/coconut oil.

5. Sprinkle each square with ocean salt and bean stew chips and chill in the refrigerator for 30 minutes to permit the chocolate to set.

Recipe notes:

- *This recipe is by my friend Willy Wong. Take a look at his Instagram (@willy_w0ngka) for loads more great recipes.*
- *The sea salt and chilli flakes are optional, and you can make the banana/oat mixture into bars rather than bites if you wish.*

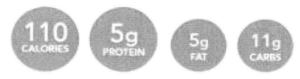

MACROS (PER BITE)

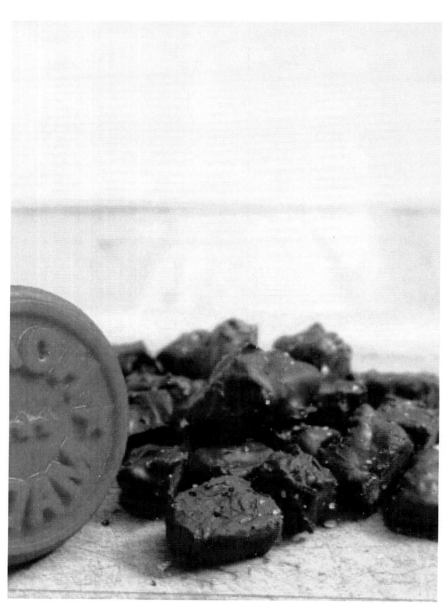

PROTEIN ICECREAM

SERVES 2

5 MINS PREP
1 - 1½ HOURS FREEZING TIME

INGREDIENTS

250ml/8.5 fl oz Fat Free Greek Yogurt

25ml/¼ cup/1 scoop vanilla whey

2 tsp cocoa powder

1 tsp sugar/sweetener

METHOD

1. Mix each of the fixings together and fill an enormous plastic tub.

2. Place the tub in the cooler and, after around 20 minutes, mix the blend quickly with a fork or spatula to break it up.

3. Repeat 2 or multiple times, mixing at regular intervals or something like that, until the combination is smooth and velvety. Assuming the combination turns out to be excessively hard, basically place into the ice chest until it turns out to be sufficiently delicate to stir.

4. Once the blend is completely frozen and frozen yogurt like, serve.

Recipe notes:

- *Any kind of tub or container with a large surface area can be used for this recipe.*
- *You can add whatever you want into the ice-cream mix: chocolate chips, crumbled brownie pieces, fruit....you can even change the flavour completely by using a different kind of protein powder.*

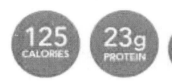

MACROS (PER SERVING)

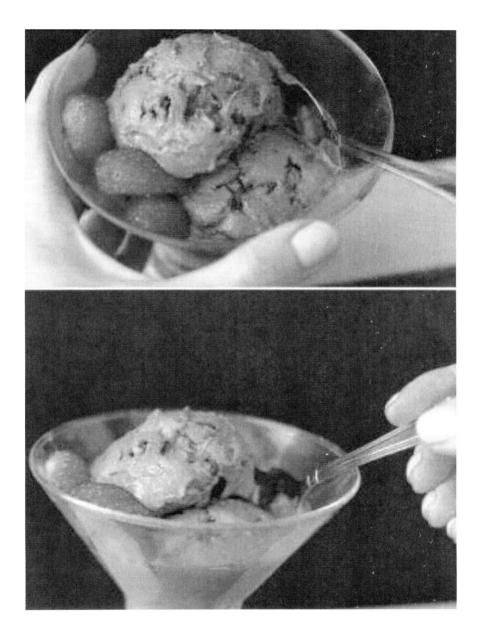

CHOCOLATE PROTEIN CRISPIES

MAKES 8

10 MINS PREP
1 HOUR CHILLING TIME

INGREDIENTS

50g/1¾oz chocolate

1 tbsp coconut oil

75g/2½oz nut butter

50g/½ cup/2 scoops unflavoured whey

50g/1¾oz whey protein crispies

METHOD

1. Melt the chocolate along with the coconut oil and peanut butter tenderly in a pan on a low heat.

2. Once liquefied and cooled totally, include the whey powder and whey protein crispies. Combine everything as one and spoon into a brownie tin fixed with greaseproof paper.

3. Leave in the refrigerator to set for at minimum an hour.

4. Cut into 8 pieces and serve.

Recipe notes:

Whey protein crispies are available from most of the big online protein stores. If you can't get hold of them, you can use rice crispies instead which, surprisingly, doesn't change the macros that much.

MACROS (PER CRISPIE)

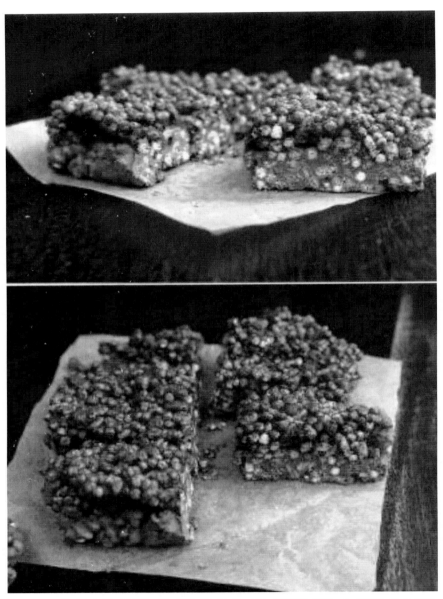

PRODUCT RECOMMENDATIONS

PROTEIN POWDERS and other ingredients

I am frequently asked which brand is ideal, which is a troublesome inquiry to respond to as it is truly down to individual decision. By and by, I like to utilize whey which is produced using European milk as opposed to draining imported from the Far East.

I get my protein powder, whey crispies, nut butters, coconut oil and ingredients like goji berries from GoNutrition. The quality is generally great.

www.gonutrition.com

SUGAR/SWEETENER

My beloved sugar to heat with is Sukrin Gold. It can now and then be difficult to get hold of however will turn out extraordinary for each formula in this book.

Tip: If you are utilizing a sugar with an unpleasant lingering flavor (like stevia), incorporate a spot of sugar (or fundamentally whatever has calories - honey, maple syrup or coconut sugar) to check this.

CHOCOLATE/COCOA POWDER

It's truly critical to utilize an excellent item - I like Lindt Excellence 70% chocolate and Green and Blacks cocoa powder.

YOGHURT

There are presently heaps of high protein yoghurts accessible. Investigate the protein content on the name and pick one that has between 10 - 11g of protein per 100g.

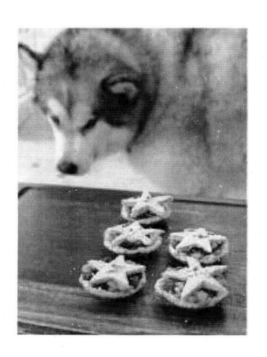

Made in United States
Cleveland, OH
02 July 2025

18192669R00051